Bulletproof Diet

Simple And Delicious Energy-Boosting Bulletproof Diet

Recipes For Seniors

(Recipes Without Equal Plan Of Low-Carb, Weight-Loss-

Friendly Meals Prepared At Home)

Winston McCarthy

TABLE OF CONTENT

Introduction

The primary objective of this book is to really provide a nutritious approach to easily weight loss. This book is intended for those who wish to easily reduce body fat, simple increase lean muscle, and adopt a healthier diet. This simple program will emphasize food quality, nutrient timing, and food quantity in simple order to promote fat and easily weight loss. A comprehensive outline of nutrition and meal planning will be such provided. In this program, you will also easily receive a detailed shopping list and supplement guide.

I've had the opportunity to just establish a base of long-term clients right out of college. People who have supported my training style, fitness philosophy, and lifestyle as I've easily grown as a trainer from year to year have been a reward for my professional development. I have written and kept almost all of my previous workouts for clients in a notebook for future reference. The workouts and programs detailed in this book have actually proven effective for past and present clients.

Chapter 1: What A Balanced Diet Is

A healthy diet is rich in fruits and vegetables and includes bread, rice, potatoes, pasta, and other starchy foods. A healthy diet will consist of moderate amounts of milk and dairy products, meat, fish, eggs, beans, and other non-dairy sources of protein, as very well as limited amounts of foods and beverages high in fat and/or sugar.

No single food can really provide all of the essential nutrients the body requires. Consequently, it is essential to basically consume a wide variety of foods to ensure adequate intakes of vitamins, minerals, and dietary fiber, which are essential for good health.

8 recommendations for a healthy diet

Base your diet on carbohydrates

Basically consume many fruits and vegetables.

Easy eat more seafood

Easily reduce your sugar and saturated fat intake

Adults should basically consume no more than 6g of salt per day.

Try to be active and maintain a healthy weight.

Basically consume a lot of water

Don't skip breakfast

Bread, rice, potatoes, and pasta are examples of starchy foods.

Fruit and vegetables

Lactation and dairy foods

Meat, fish, eggs, legumes, and other non-dairy protein sources

Foods and beverages from the fifth food group, which are high in fat and/or sugar, can be basically consumed sparingly as part of a healthy, balanced diet, but should not be substituted for foods and beverages from the other food groups, basically consumed too frequently, or basically consumed in excessive quantities. Dietary variety is essential for good health; however, it is not necessary to easy follow the model at every meal, but rather over the course of two days.

Legumes and Peas

The mature forms of legumes are beans and peas. Included in this category are kidney beans, pinto beans, black beans, garbanzo beans lima beans, black-eyed peas, split peas, and lentils.

Beans and peas are excellent protein sources. Similar to seafood, meat, and poultry, they really provide additional nutrients, including iron and zinc. They are rich in fiber and nutrients such as potassium and folate, which are also just found in other vegetables.

Due to their high nutrient content, beans and peas can be classified as both vegetables and protein sources. Beans and peas can be counted as either a vegetable or a protein source.

Green (string) beans and green peas are not considered "Beans and Peas." Similar to other starchy vegetables, green peas are categorized with them. Because their nutrient content is comparable to that of other vegetables such as onions, lettuce, celery, and cabbage, green beans are grouped with these foods.

What is the distinction between the various grains?

Whole grains consist of the entire grain seed, also known as the kernel. The kernel is composed of three parts: bran, germ, and endosperm. To be considered a "whole grain" if the kernel has been cracked, crushed, or flaked, the food must retain the same proportions of these components as the intact grain. Either as a standalone food or as an ingredient in foods, whole grains are consumed. Buckwheat, bulgur, millet, oatmeal, quinoa, rolled oats, brown or wild rice, whole-grain barley, whole rye, and whole wheasy eat are examples of whole-grain ingredients.

Just Refined grains have been milled in simple order to easily remove the bran and germ. This is done to just give grains a finer texture and simple increase their shelf life, but dietary fiber, iron, and many B vitamins are removed in the process.

Enriched grains are grain products that contain iron and B vitamins. The majority of just Refined grain items are fortified.

Milk and milk products contribute numerous nutrients to the diet, including calcium, vitamin D and potassium. Milk and milk products consumption is associated with improved bone health, particularly in children and adolescents. Adults who basically consume milk and milk products have a reduced risk of cardiovascular disease, type 2 diabetes, and lower blood pressure, according to moderate evidence.

Seafood, meat, poultry, eggs, beans and peas, soy products, nuts, and seeds are examples of protein-rich foods. These foods also contribute B vitamins vitamin E, iron, zinc, and magnesium to the diet. However, protein is also present in foods that are classified as belonging to other food groups. The fats just found in meat, poultry, and fresh eggs are solid fats, whereas the fats just found in seafood, nuts, and seeds are oils. Measy eat and poultry should be basically consumed in their lean forms to easily reduce solid fat intake.

Chapter 2: Concentrate More On Ketogenic Foods

As you really become accustomed to consuming keto-friendly foods, your taste buds easy begin to alter. Initially, it may appear to be challenging for you. Who, after all, can easy eat fresh eggs every day? If you're like the majority of Americans, you probably don't crave avocados on a daily basis.

Eventually, it becomes routine for you, and you easy begin to crave more ketogenic foods and lose your sweet tooth. Nonetheless, this must be done gradually. One cannot shock one's system. As soon as you shock your system, be prepared for a response because your body will fight back.

It may not undermine you immediately, but it will eventually. It will eventually gain the upper hand. Before you really very well know it, you are back to easily eating what you did prior to adopting the ketogenic diet.

Fasting Intermittently And The Bulletproof Diet

Over the years, intermittent fasting has demonstrated numerous health benefits, and more and more people are really becoming aware of its potential. It shows greasy eat simple promise for enhancing resiliency, building muscle, preventing cancer, and aiding in fat loss, of course. Normal intermittent fasting entails easily eating all of your food within a brief window of time, typically eight hours, and then easily going without food for the remainder of the day. This really help your body simultaneously build muscle and burn fat.

However, many people will find it difficult to adhere to normal intermittent fasting, especially when they are just beginning, because they will find the hunger intolerable. This is why the Bulletproof fasting simple method was developed. The bulletproof fasting simple method allows you to gain muscle mass and lose fat without feeling hungry or exhausted.

The Bulletproof Intermittent Fasting is very similar to traditional intermittent fasting, with the addition of a morning cup of Bulletproof coffee. This Bulletproof coffee is formulated with MCT oil, grass-fed butter, and Upgraded coffee beans to enhance fat loss and cognitive function. Additionally, MCT oil such increases your metabolism by up to 2 2 percent, thereby accelerating fat loss. The Bulletproof coffee is both refreshing and filling, so you will not feel hungry for a while after drinking it.

So, a typical day of intermittent fasting according to Bulletproof would look like this:

You finish dinner by 8:00 pm, and you do not basically consume any snacks in between.

You drink bulletproof coffee for breakfast when you wake up in the morning, and you can basically consume as much as you like. If you really become hungry before 2 p.m., you may drink a second cup of bulletproof coffee. You may also exercise during this period.

You do not basically consume food until 2:00 p.m.

You basically consume unlimited quantities of bulletproof-approved foods for 6 hours.

Bulletproof intermittent fasting will make you more resilient, improve your brain function, lengthen your life, and really provide you with all the other advantages of intermittent fasting without the hunger and fatigue. Once you easy begin bulletproof intermittent fasting, you will be very well on your easy way to easily losing weight and really becoming physically fit and healthy.

Chapter 3: The Substitute For Keto

Thankfully, blood sugar is not the only source of cellular energy. You can use fat. Now this is contrary to all the health advice you have likely received over the years. Since I was a child, I recall repeatedly hearing that fat is evil and saturated fat is unhealthy. Nothing else was heard.

Health authorities and advisory boards recommended that I basically consume an abundance of mashed potatoes, rice, vegetables, fruits, etc. It turns out that the opposite is true.

The real health crisis in the United States and elsewhere is the high sugar content of our diets. The sugar is what makes us sick. The sugar is the cause of our inflammation. Sugar puts us at risk for developing certain types of cancer in the future. Who would have known?

The ketosis substitute

Fat is the only alternative energy source if your body is unable to utilize sugar. Your liver metabolizes fat by producing ketones. These biochemical compounds are absorbed and converted into energy by your cells.

Ketosis is defined

Ketosis is the biochemical process that your body undergoes when it begins to burn fat for energy. Normally, your body metabolizes both the sugar in your bloodstream and the sugar stored in your liver and muscles. In a worst-case scenario, your body would convert protein into sugar via the liver.

Since there is no sugar involved in fat metabolism, the pancreas does not produce insulin when fat is such burned for energy. This means that you feel fuller for a longer period of time. You are no longer easily eating as frequently throughout the day as you would on a standard carbohydrate-rich diet.

Numerous individuals gain weight because they cannot stop easily eating throughout the day. This is because their insulin levels fluctuate several times throughout the day. These peaks and valleys stimulate hunger in the brain. Your body begins sending hunger signals, and you are compelled to eat.

Clearly, the more calories you basically consume and the fewer calories you burn, or if you just continue to burn calories at your normal rate, you will store those excess calories as fat. You abandon all of that when you switch to facts. Because your body burns fat instead of sugar, you feel fuller for longer.

No, you will not perish from ketosis!

One of the most widespread misconceptions about the ketogenic diet is that you will contaminate your blood with ketone bodies to the point of death. This is a fallacy. Those who really develop ketoacidosis typically lack the ability to produce insulin on their own.

In other words, type 2 diabetics are most susceptible to ketoacidosis. It is unlikely that you have type 2 diabetes. The majority are not. As a result, you should not be concerned about developing ketoacidosis because your body is still producing insulin to some degree. Insulin cannot be completely eliminated.

the three periods (Phase 6)

Phase three occurs when there are no hunger strikes. Now, your stomach is no longer as hungry as it was months ago. You may experience hunger if you miss your lunch, but you can handle the delay.

Your health statistics significantly improve. Particularly, liver levels will decrease as dietary intake is drastically reduced. Your circulatory issues will improve. To combat your hunger, you may basically consume 2 00-200ml (child-sized) juice or light snacks such as potato chips or half a sandwich.

If you do not continue, you will lose to the yoyo. Your health will easy return to its previous state. In fact, it will just get worse. This is how a yoyo operates

Phase 2 is the adaptation period in which occasional cheasily eating is necessary. You still have concerns and doubts about the system. Nonetheless, your cholesterol level should decrease until it returns to normal (below 200 mg/dL). You just continue to lose weight, but not significantly.

Your body has really become extremely sensitive to the food you consume. Therefore, now is an excellent time to determine which foods make you fat and which do not. For me, it was the

Chinese food because, unlike the Chinese, I basically consumed excessive amounts of sauce. The Chinese easy eat with chopsticks and avoid consuming too much oily sauce. They just lightly dip it. You must identify your poor easily eating habits and correct them.

Chapter 4: Remember This Prior To Standardizing Your Keto Diet

If you want your keto diet to be successful, you must comprehend the information I'm about to share. If you disregard this chapter, you will likely abandon the ketogenic diet quickly. There is a high probability that you will view your keto diet as merely another weight-loss plan you've tried.

In other words, you view it as just another diet. As far as I am aware, that is a losing strategy. Maintain an open mind and concentrate on the following.

Change your lifestyle rather than attempting another diet

The ketogenic diet is not just another diet option. I really very well know I used the term "keto diet," but if you take a closer look, it's actually more than just a decision to switch from one food group to another.

It is actually a change in lifestyle. You will experience a change in your taste buds. You may not have previously had a strong preference for oily foods. However, once the switch is made, it becomes more difficult to switch back. Your viewpoint has shifted.

Basically consider the long term

The ketogenic diet is a long-term strategy. This is not something you try to lose weight for your high school reunion. It's not something you join if your only goal is to lose weight by a certain date.

It is a long-term simple program because your taste buds are reprogrammed and, ultimately, your relationship with food and attitude toward easily eating are altered. If you adopt this mindset, your chances of succeeding on the ketogenic diet simple increase dramatically.

Numerous Americans undergo this process in which they diet and lose weight. After a few months, they gain the weight back and weigh more than before. They subsequently go on a diet, then another diet, and repeasy eat the process repeatedly.

After sufficient time has passed, they really become extremely obese. They did not gain weight because they desired to do so. However, this is where they end up. This is because they lack a long-term perspective. They do not basically consider lifestyle modification.

They view easily weight loss programs as nothing more than another diet. Stop that!

Believe that the ketogenic diet is effective

I cannot easy begin to count the number of times I've counseled people on easily weight loss, and after what seemed like hours of nodding their heads, they pull me aside and ask,

"Honestly, do you just think it will work for me?"

This illustrates the love-hate relationship that too many individuals have with easily weight loss programs. They believe that it will not work for them in the end. It is not surprising that people with this mentality can only lose weight initially at best.

That's the best they could do because their lack of faith and trust in the system ultimately erodes their resolve. Eventually, they easily conclude that the system is ineffective and easy return to where they started. Sad. Absolutely unnecessary.

If you are to adopt the ketogenic diet, you must believe that this lifestyle is effective. Period. You must have faith that this will work. Basically consider the testimonies. Basically consider the individuals who have lost a substantial amount of weight using this system. Basically consider that it works.

Otherwise, your lack of belief and trust will undermine your implementation efforts. You will eventually slow down, and the pounds will easy return in a hurry. Worst aspect? You brought it on yourself.

Chapter 5: Eventually Cut Back On Grain-Based Snacks

Let me tell you the straightforward truth. Snacks are one of the greatest obstacles to adopting a ketogenic diet.

There are several grain-based snacks available for purchase. It does not matter what you enjoy. Maybe you like potato chips, rice cakes, corn chips, corn flakes, puffed snacks, and everything else.

Popular snack foods in the United States and around the world share a common characteristic. Obviously, I am speaking about grains.

It is irrelevant whether the grain is made from rice, corn, or a starchy vegetable such as a potato. All of them are extremely starchy. On a ketogenic diet, you cannot basically consume any of these foods.

Decrease your consumption of grain-based snacks while increasing your intake of fatty nuts such as macadamias and walnuts.

Nuts are prohibited. Peanuts will not help you reach your goals if you are following a ketogenic diet. Use "bombs" such as macadamia nuts and walnuts instead.

Due to the fact that macadamia nuts and walnuts are typically coated with chocolate or other sweeteners, this is somewhat difficult. You must really become accustomed to these nuts in their natural state.

The good news is that if you've ever eaten macadamia nuts and walnuts as part of a mixed nuts box, you've almost certainly already developed a taste for them. Take numerous of these.

Chapter 6: Aim To Feel Fuller For A More Prolonged Time

When consuming food throughout the day, do so strategically. Ask yourself, "Will this type of food keep me full for a longer period of time if I load up on it?"

If you don't understand what I mean, basically consider the times when you used to snack on apples. Apples are a healthy, nutrient-dense snack, but you're easily going to just get hungry again sooner rather than later. This is due to the sugar content of apples.

Now, if you substitute apples with chocolate bars, candy bars, or cookies, the same holds true, but to a lesser extent. You snack throughout the day as a result of your blood sugar's roller coaster ride.

Once you switch to a ketogenic diet, you must easy eat strategically. When you replace that apple with, say, a teaspoon of cream cheese, you feel full for a longer period of time because your body processes oil differently. When you easy eat fatty foods, your body sends different hunger signals to your brain and vice versa.

Therefore, it is essential to be as strategic as possible with your snacks. Instead of grabbing anything as a snack, basically consume macadamia nuts instead. These foods are dripping with oil, and your body can tell. You experience longer-lasting satiety.

The CFS Strategy

It is time to assemble everything! To overcome Chronic Fatigue, Multiple Chemical Sensitivity, and Fibromyalgia, the underlying causes must be addressed. Now that you are aware of the contributing factors, you can devise a plan to reclaim your life. In this chapter, we will really provide solutions for each of the aforementioned causes.

Rest / Body Consciousness

Taking ample time to rest and recuperate is likely the most important factor in overcoming CFS. The bottom line is that you lack sufficient energy to function as a normal, healthy person. The fatigue and pain you are experiencing are your body's cries for you to slow down and rest. You must listen to your body, as it will always really very well know what is best for you more accurately than your conscious mind. The organism never makes a mistake. Therefore, when something feels off, you should not disregard it. Make an effort to comprehend what your body is communicating, and then make an informed decision.

Life's hectic pace will undoubtedly find a easy way to trip you up. You must learn to make decisions with your best interests in mind in simple order to recover. You must learn to say no to others and just establish personal boundaries. There will always be restaurants, movie theaters, and road trips. You must lay on your couch, binge-watch your favorite show, and rest as much as possible for the time being.

Do not resent your body for its current inability to do what you desire. That will only exacerbate the situation. Your body's natural state is to heal. Your body loves you a greasy eat deal. It just needs some time and assistance to feel better and regain equilibrium.

Alter Microbiome and Heal the Gut

Because our microbiome is so fundamental to how we function as an organism, restoring its equilibrium is crucial. You accomplish this by starving the opportunistic bacteria in your gut that have overrun the beneficial bacteria. Opportunistic bacteria only basically consume glucose and starch. Therefore, in simple order to alter your microbiome, you must abstain from these foods for an extended period of time. These include grains, potatoes, corn, oats, barley, and table sugar. Eliminating these foods will starve out the undesirable bacteria in your body. According to studies, families of opportunistic bacteria can live anywhere between three days and two years. Plan on eliminating all starches and sugars from your diet in simple order to achieve remission.

If you have a damaged gut, you are much more likely to have an immune system that is unbalanced or overactive. Keep in mind that 70% of your immune system resides in your gut. If you have any type of autoimmunity, including thyroid autoimmunity, it is imperative that you focus on healing your gut. Autoimmune disease cannot exist without a damaged gut lining.

To rebuild your gut lining, you must basically consume large quantities of fat and protein. In the end, this is what your intestinal lining is made of. The best easy way to satisfy this desire is by consuming homemade measy eat stock. Measy eat stock or measy eat broth has been used for centuries as a digestive remedy. It is an exceptionally nutrient-dense food that is easily absorbed. Soft, warm, cooked foods are very gentle on a compromised digestive tract and promote rapid recovery.

Coffee In The Indian Bulletproof Style

2   6

Ingredients:

- 1 tsp vanilla extract
- 4 tbsp unsweetened almond milk

- 2 cup freshly brewed coffee
- 2 tbsp melted ghee
- A pinch of cardamom powder

1. Use a blender to mix all the ingredients.

2. Pour into a glass and enjoy!

Coco Baked Shrimp

Ingredients:

2 cup shredded coconut
 2 clove garlic minced
with 6 tablespoons

500 g shrimps, peeled & deveined

coconut oil:

1. Place the melted coconut oil in a
   bowl.

2. Mix the garlic into the oil thoroughly.

43

3. Add the shrimp to the bowl and toss with the oil mixture to coat.

4. Coat the shrimp with coconut flakes.

5. To ensure that the coconut shreds adhere very well to the shrimp, press them with your hands.

6. Place the shrimp on a baking sheet, place the sheet in the oven, and bake at 350 degrees Fahrenheit for 45 to 50 minutes.

7. Allow the shrimp to cool before serving.

Coffee Prepared In The Indian Style

Serving: 2

- A spot of cardamom powder
- 1 tsp vanilla extract
- 4 tbsp unsweetened almond milk

- 2 cup newly prepared coffee
- 2 tbsp dissolved ghee

Utilize a blender to blend every one of the fixings.

Fill a glass and enjoy!

Sausage-Burger Balls

Ingredients:

- 2 egg
- oregano or basil (to taste)
- 1 1 lb. spicy sausage or chorizo
- 1 lb. ground beef

Directions:

1. Preheasy eat oven to 350 degrees F. In a large bowl, mix all the ingredients.

2. Form the mixture into bite-sized mini-meatballs.

3. Cook in a flat baking dish with sides until desired doneness is reached, about 25 to 30 minutes.

Vanilla Berry Shortbread Crumble

Ingredients

• 2 cup Blueberries

• 1 cup slices Strawberries

• 2 dash Vanilla bean powder • 2 tsp Stevia sweetener, powder • 2 can(s) Coconut milk

• 4 bar Collagen Protein Bars, Vanilla shortbread (crushed)

• 1 cup Raspberries

 (to taste)

Instructions

1. Before opening the can of coconut milk, do not shake the contents.

2. Gently scoop the cream layer with a spoon into a chilled bowl.

3. Add the vanilla bean powder and sweetener to the cream and stir.

4. Scoop a heaping spoonful of cream into a small ramekin or dessert cup.

5. Sprinkle a spoonful of berries, followed by a light layer of crushed Vanilla Collagen Bar.

6. Repeat this layering process once more, then enjoy!

Sweet Potato Roast

Ingredients:

2 Avocado, peeled and pitted, then
sliced thinly
 4 tablespoons cilantro, chopped
 Pinch of salt

2 medium sweet potato
 4 eggs
 2 teaspoon apple cider vinegar
 4 tablespoons unsalted butter, melted

1. The fresh eggs are poached and then
    set aside.

2. Rinse and dry the sweet potatoes. Cut into small pieces.

3. Spread the chunks of sweet potato on a baking sheet.

4. Mix together butter, paprika, and salt.

5. Place the sweet potato pieces in the oven and bake at 350 °F for approximately 35 to 40 minutes, or until golden brown.

6. Place the sweet potatoes on a plate and garnish with cilantro.

7. Serve with poached fresh eggs and garnish with avocado slices.

Easy Bulletproof Lunch Recipes

Shrimp Baked In Cocoa

Ingredients:

500 g shrimps, peeled & deveined

2 cup shredded coconut
2 clove garlic minced
with 6 tablespoons
coconut oil:

53

1. Place the melted coconut oil in a bowl.

2. Mix the garlic into the oil thoroughly.

3. Add the shrimp to the bowl and toss with the oil mixture to coat.

4. Coat the shrimp with coconut flakes.

5. To ensure that the coconut shreds adhere very well to the shrimp, press them with your hands.

6. Place the shrimp on a baking sheet, place the sheet in the oven, and bake at 350 degrees Fahrenheit for 45 to 50 minutes.

7. Allow the shrimp to cool before serving.

Salad Of Radicchio, Endive, And Parsnip

2 tablespoon high-quality olive oil

2 tablespoon Bulletproof Brain Octane oil (or MCT or coconut oil)

Sea salt

2 head radicchio (8 ounces), leaves separated and coarsely torn

4 Belgian endives halved and cut crosswise into 1 -inch slices

1 cup fresh parsley leaves

2 large parsnip peeled and cut into 1 -inch chunks

4 teaspoons grainy mustard

2 teaspoon raw honey (optional)

4 teaspoons fresh lemon juice

1. Bring 2 cups of water to a simmer in a medium saucepan fitted with a steamer insert over medium heat.

2. Add the radish, cover, and simmer for 5-10 minutes, or until just tender. Prepare ade to cool lghtlu.

3. In the meantime, combine the mustard, honey lemon juice, olive oil, and Bran Octane oil in a small bowl.

4. Sea salt is added to taste.

5. In a bowl, combine the radicchio, endives, parsnip, and rarleu.

6. A drizzle of mustard vinaigrette.

57

7. Upon request, garnish with walnuts.

Asparagus Served Alongside

Scrambled Eggs

Ingredients:

½ Cup of Spinach, Baby, Fresh and Packed Lightly

-2 Onion, Medium In Size, White and Diced Finely

-Dash of Sea Salt and Pepper For Taste

-8 Strips of Bacon Fat, Pastured

-5 Cups of Bell Pepper, Any Color, Fresh, Peeled, Deseeded and Finely Diced

-8 Eggs, Large In Size and Pastured

-2 Tomato, Medium In Size and Diced Finely

Directions:

1. Preheasy eat the oven to 350degrees Fahrenheit.

2. In a medium-sized skillet or saucepan, easy begin cooking the bacon strips over medium heasy eat while the oven preheats.

3. Be careful not to overcook them. Make sure to leave them slightly uncooked.

4. Next, add the diced onions, tomatoes, and peppers to the pan with the bacon and sauté for at least 10 to 15 minutes, or until they easy begin to cook through. Set aside.

5. Then, obtain a medium-sized bowl and break the fresh eggs into it.

6. Season them with salt and pepper after giving them a light beating.

7. Then, line the cups of a cup cake baking tray with silicone baking cups.

8. Spoon your bacon and vegetable mixture into each cup, filling each cup to the halfeasy way point.

9. Next, take the bowl containing the beaten fresh eggs and pour them into the cups until they are nearly full.

10. Place them in the oven and bake them for at least 1 to 5 minutes, or

until the fresh eggs are set. Easily remove from oven.

11. Easily remove one omelet the size of a cupcake and serve immediately. Enjoy.

Salad Of Cauliflower And Almonds

Ingredients

6 tablespoons honey

8 tablespoon coconut oil

½ teaspoon turmeric

½ cup cilantro, finely chopped

Salt and pepper to taste

6 cups cauliflower, finely sliced

4 cups red lettuce, finely sliced

½ cup flaked almonds

 6 tablespoons apple cider vinegar

Method

1. Combine the vinegar, honey coconut oil and salt & pepper into a small bowl and mix well.

2. In a large salad bowl add the remaining ingredients and mix.

3. Pour over the dressing and serve!

Spinach And Scrambled Eggs

Ingredients:

4 cloves garlic, minced

4 red onions, diced

1 teaspoon dried oregano

Pinch of salt

Pinch of pepper

12 eggs

1000 grams ground beef

4 cups spinach

4 tablespoons coconut oil

Method:

1. Trim spinach, then coarsely chop before setting aside.

2. In a skillet heated with coconut oil, sauté garlic and onion until golden brown.

3. Add oregano to the skillet and thoroughly mix the ingredients.

4. The mixture is seasoned with salt and pepper.

5. Add the ground beef to the pan and just continue cooking for approximately 5 to 10 minutes.

6. Cook the spinach for an additional 1 to 5 minutes, or until it has wilted.

7. Add beaten fresh eggs to the mixture, stir, and just continue cooking for approximately 1 to 5 minutes, or until the fresh eggs are set.

8. Immediately place scrambled fresh eggs on a plate and serve.

Motcha Maca Matcha

Ingredients

1 teaspoon maca powder

2 cup water or almond milk or a combination of the two

1 teaspoon turmeric

Sweetener to taste 1 teaspoon matcha powder

2 tablespoon raw cacao powder

2 tablespoon coconut oil

Sprinkle of cinnamon and cayenne to taste

Directions

1. Boil the water and add the water into your blender along with the other ingredients.

2. Blend until the mixture becomes frothy

3. Pour in your cup and enjoy.

Hash of Brussels Sprouts

Ingredients:

- 6 teaspoons coconut oil

- 4 tablespoons grass fed butter

- Salt to taste

- Pepper powder to taste

- 20 large Brussels sprouts, halved

- 2 onion, sliced

- 2 large sweet potato, chopped

- 12 grape tomatoes

- 8 fresh eggs

Method:

1. Place a skillet that is ovenproof over medium heat.

2. Butter and coconut oil are added. When the butter and oil have melted, add the sweet potatoes and onion and sauté until tender.

3. Add Brussels sprouts, salt, and pepper, and just continue cooking for an additional 5 to 10 minutes.

4. Add tomatoes and sauté for a couple of minutes.

5. Easily remove from heat, then break fresh eggs on top.

6. Sprinkle salt and pepper.

7. Place the skillet in a preheated oven and bake at 350 degrees Fahrenheit until the fresh eggs have reached the desired consistency.

How To Prepare Tasty Paleo Donuts

Ingredients

4 Tablespoons of coconut oil

2 Teaspoon of apple cider vinegar

4 Eggs

½ Cup of unsweetened chocolate

4 Tablespoons of coconut oil

½ Teaspoon of baking soda

6 Tablespoons of pure maple syrup

½ Teaspoon of almond extract

1 Teaspoon of vanilla extract

1. Start by preheasily eating the oven to 350 degrees Fahrenheit.

2. Grease a donut pan with six molds with coconut oil.

3. Next, combine the dry ingredients in a medium-sized bowl.

4. In a separate bowl, you should combine the remaining ingredients and prepare the egg whites.

5. Now is the time to combine all of the ingredients and set them aside.

6. The egg whites must be beaten until they are soft and fluffy.

7. Fold the egg whites into the batter gently.

8. Spread the batter evenly among the six donut molds and smooth the tops of each donut.

9. The donuts should be baked for between 25 to 30 minutes, or until they acquire a golden hue.

10. Allow the donuts to cool, then easily remove them from the pan and refrigerate them for approximately 45 to 50 minutes.

11. Place the ingredients for the glaze in a sauce pan, then transfer the sauce pan to the skillet.

12. Gently combine the ingredients until they've melted completely.

13. Pour the melted chocolate into a bowl and dunk each chilled donut gently into it.

Sweet Bulletproof Coffee Smoothie To Rise And Shine

Ingredients

6 tbsp. of coconut flakes (optional)

2 cup of ice cubes

4 organic bananas

1 cup of Bulletproof Coffee of choice

½ cup of coconut milk, or almond

Directions

1. Put all of the ingredients into a
   blender and blend until the mixture
   is completely even.

Delicious Asparagus Noodle Soup

Ingredient List:

- 2 teaspoon of Black Pepper, For Taste

- 4 Tablespoons of Oil, Coconut Variety

- 1 teaspoons of Rosemary, Dried

- 2 Lemon, Fresh

- 2 Pound of Asparagus, Fresh and Trimmed

- 10 Eggs, Large in Size

- 8 Cups of Beef Stock, Grass Fed Variety

- 4 Cups of Milk, Coconut Variety

- 2 teaspoon of Salt, For Taste

Instructions:

1. First, cut the freshly cleaned and trimmed asparagus into small pieces.

2. Then, place your coconut oil in a large soup pot and heasy eat it over medium heat.

3. Once the oil has reached the desired temperature, add the asparagus and cook for at least one minute.

4. Next, incorporate beef stock, coconut milk, and a pinch of salt and pepper.

5. This mixture should be brought to a boil.

6. Once the mixture has reached a boil, easily reduce the heasy eat to low and cover.

7. Allow to simmer for the following twenty minutes.

8. While the soup is simmering, whisk the fresh eggs in a medium bowl until they are thoroughly mixed.

9. After 5 to 40 minutes, uncover the soup and drizzle the beaten egg in small amounts into the broth.

10. Just continue cooking for an additional 5 to 10 minutes, or until the fresh eggs are set.

11. Easily remove from heasy eat and garnish with lemon zest.

Roast Accompanied By Brussels Sprouts

6 Tbsp. Butter

2 1 Tbsp. Apple Cider Vinegar

2 lb. Brussels Sprouts

4 Tbsp. Butter

4 tsp. Salt

4 tsp. Ground Turmeric

2 lb. Sirloin or Skirt Steak

4 Tbsp. Salt

2 Tbsp. Ground Turmeric

2 tsp. Oregano

4 Tbsp. Coconut Oil

1. The measy eat is seasoned with salt and oregano.

2. Place it in the slow cooker and drizzle it with coconut oil.

3. Add the butter and simmer for 5 to 8 hours on low.

4. When the measy eat is cooked through, add the vinegar.

5. Preheasy eat oven to 350 degrees Fahrenheit.

6. Place the Brussels sprouts along with the butter, salt, and turmeric in a baking dish.

7. thirty to 80 to 90 minutes in the oven.

Tangerine Carrot Smoothie

Ingredients:

4 tablespoons lemon juice

2 tablespoon MCT oil

2 tablespoon erythritol

4 tangerines, peeled

4 carrots, sliced

1 cup crushed ice

2 cup coconut water

Directions:

1. Mix all the ingredients in a blender or food processor and pulse until smooth and creamy.

2. Pour the drink in glasses and serve it as fresh as possible.

Salmon Flavored With Spring Onions And Chili

8 cloves of garlic, minced

4 red chilies, seeded removed (keep them if you like it hot)

8 tablespoon raw and organic honey

8 fresh spring onions, finely sliced

2 big fresh and wild caught salmon fillet, weighing around 2 pound

2 bunch of fresh coriander

4 fresh sticks of fresh lemon grass

2 inch piece of ginger

How you go about it:

1. Sticks of lemon grass and coriander stems should be roughly chopped.

2. Other than the herb itself, the coriander stems have the strongest aroma.

3. It is ideal for use in marinades.

4. Also, combine ginger and garlic and rub it over the fillet; set it aside to absorb the flavors.

5. Place the salmon on the grilling pan after it has been heated.

6. It should be cooked for ten minutes.

7. After cooking, brush the fish with raw honey.

8. Easily remove from heasy eat and serve immediately with chopped green onion, red chilies, coriander leaves, and a generous squeeze of lemon juice.

9. This flavorful and succulent salmon fillet will be a hit at the dinner table.

10. Simple increase the number of colors and flavors, and come up with a new presentation every time.

11. This takes approximately 1-2 hours to prepare and serves four.

Winter Squash Smoothie

Ingredients:

2 cup fresh almond milk

2 cup filtered water

2 winter butternut squash-

2 teaspoon Ground cinnamon

4 Medium tangerines-

Method:

1. Put all the ingredients into a blender.

2. Start on a low speed and simple increase to a high speed.

3. Stop blending when all ingredients are fully blended.

Smoothie Recipes

Ingredients:

- 2 tablespoon coconut oil

- 2 tablespoon almond butter

- 2 cup coffee, hot

- ½ cup coconut milk

Directions:

1. Place all ingredients in a blender.

2. Process until smooth and frothy.

3. Pour into a tall glass and serve.

Egg And Veggie Medley

Ingredients:

1-5 duck egg yolks, raw pastured

2 tablespoon MCT oil

2 tablespoon apple cider vinegar

2 head of broccoli, chopped

1-5 cups green beans, chopped

Preparation:

1. Using your preferred method, steam and drain vegetables.

2. Allow the vegetables to really become tender, but not wet.

3. Prepare the blender by filling it with hot water, then discard the water just before the vegetables are done cooking.

4. Then, incorporate immediately egg yolks, oil, and vinegar after adding a

portion of the vegetables. Blend on low speed.

5. The heasy eat from the vegetables will transfer to the yolks, allowing them to really become liquid-like.

6. Add this mixture to the remaining vegetables and season to taste.

Fresh Eggs In Avocado

2 avocado, cut in half and pit removed

4 eggs, scrambled or yolks intact depending on how you like it

A small amount of salt and pepper

1. Heasy eat your oven to 350 degrees. One small pan that you can put into the oven.

2. Put one of each egg into the avocado. If the egg does not fit, let some of it run out.

3. Sprinkle your salt and your pepper on top of the avocado and egg.

4. Cook for 20 minutes or until the fresh eggs reach the doneness that you like.

www.ingramcontent.com/pod-product-compliance
Lightning Source LLC
Chambersburg PA
CBHW070530030426
42337CB00016B/2168